The Glucose Innovation:

How Understanding and Managing Your Blood Sugar Can Transform Your Health.

Unlocking the Secrets to Optimal Health, Energy, and Longevity
Through Smart Glucose Management

BY

Jennifer Danielson

TABLE OF CONTENT

INTRODUCTION

The Glucose Innovation is a movement aimed at better comprehending and handling blood sugar levels. Glycemic control has become increasingly important in the prevention and management of chronic conditions such as diabetes, cardiovascular disease, obesity, and cognitive decline in recent years, according to research. Recognizing the role of glucose in the body and implementing strategies to manage blood sugar levels through diet, exercise, and lifestyle changes are all part of the Glucose Revolution

.

In this book, we will go over the Glucose Innovation concept in depth and explain how understanding and managing your blood sugar levels can transform your health. We will look at the science of glucose metabolism and the consequences of poor glucose metabolism. The effects of glucose management on health, energy, and longevity. We will also discuss blood sugar management strategies, such as dietary approaches, exercise and physical activity, lifestyle changes, and nutritional supplements. We will offer practical advice on how to implement a glucose management plan, set goals, track progress, and stay motivated and consistent.

The Glucose Innovation offers a powerful approach to optimal health, whether you want to prevent chronic disease, improve athletic performance, or simply feel better and more energetic in your daily life. By the end of this book, you will have a thorough understanding of the significance of glucose management, as well as the tools necessary to take charge of your health and well-being.

CHAPTER 1

What exactly is the Glucose Innovation?

The Glucose Innovation refers to the movement toward better understanding and management of blood sugar levels for optimal health. It is the notion that controlling glucose levels through diet, exercise, and lifestyle changes can have a significant impact on overall health and well-being. Recognizing the importance of glycemic control in preventing and managing chronic conditions such as diabetes, cardiovascular disease, obesity, and cognitive decline is part of the Glucose Innovation. Individuals can unlock the secrets to optimal health, energy, and longevity by understanding the role of glucose in the body and implementing strategies to manage blood sugar levels. The Sugar Revolution represents a shift toward preventive health care and is based on the most recent scientific research on glucose metabolism and its impact on health.

Smart glucose management is critical for overall health, energy, and longevity. Because glucose is the primary source of fuel for the body's cells, proper glucose management is critical for overall health, energy, and longevity. Glucose is derived from the foods we consume and converted into energy via a process known as cellular respiration.

However, if glucose levels are not properly managed, they can lead to several health issues such as diabetes, obesity, and cardiovascular disease. High blood sugar levels can also cause inflammation and oxidative stress, both of which can harm cells and hasten aging. Maintaining stable blood sugar levels, on the other hand, through smart glucose management, can provide numerous benefits. It can, for example, aid in energy regulation, mental clarity and focus, healthy weight management, and the prevention of chronic diseases.

Smart glucose management entails several strategies, including:

1. Consuming a well-balanced diet rich in carbohydrates, protein, and healthy fats.

2. Refrain from sugary and processed foods, which can cause blood sugar spikes. Including physical activity in your daily routine to improve insulin sensitivity and muscle glucose uptake.

3. Regularly check blood sugar levels, especially for diabetics.

4. Using stress-reduction techniques such as meditation or mindfulness to reduce stress hormones that can raise blood sugar levels.

CHAPTER 2:

Glucose Basics

Glucose is a type of sugar that serves as the primary source of energy for the cells in the body. It is a simple carbohydrate found in a variety of foods such as fruits, vegetables, and grains. When we eat carbohydrates, our bodies convert them into glucose, which is then transported to our cells via the bloodstream. Once inside the cells, glucose is used to generate energy via a process known as cellular respiration. Insulin, a hormone produced by the pancreas, is critical in regulating blood glucose levels. It facilitates the entry of glucose into cells and signals the liver to store excess glucose as glycogen. When blood glucose levels fall, another hormone called glucagon signals the liver to break down glycogen and reintroduce glucose into the bloodstream.

Abnormal glucose levels can cause health issues. Over time, high blood glucose levels can damage blood vessels and organs, leading to complications such as cardiovascular disease, kidney disease, and nerve damage. Low blood glucose levels, on the other hand, can cause symptoms such as weakness, confusion, and even loss of consciousness.

Insulin's Role in Blood Sugar Regulation

Insulin is a hormone produced with the aid of using the pancreas that performs an critical position in blood sugar regulation. When you eat something, your body breaks it down into glucose, which is then absorbed into your bloodstream. Your pancreas releases insulin into your bloodstream as your blood sugar levels rise.Insulin performs numerous roles in blood sugar regulation. It benefits your cells to absorb glucose from the bloodstream and use it for energy or store it for later use.

Insulin also instructs the liver to absorb glucose and convert it to glycogen, a stored form of glucose that can be released when blood sugar levels fall. Diabetes occurs when the body either fails to produce enough insulin (type 1 diabetes) or cannot utilize the insulin that is produced (type 2 diabetes). This can result in high blood sugar levels, which can damage organs and tissues all over the body over time. Diabetes patients may require insulin shots or other treatments to help regulate their blood sugar levels. Overall, insulin is important in blood sugar regulation because it helps to transport glucose from the bloodstream into cells, where it can be used for energy or stored for later use.

Factors Influencing Blood Sugar Levels

Several factors can influence blood sugar levels, including:

1. Diet: The types and amounts of food you eat can have a significant impact on your blood sugar levels. Carbohydrate and sugar-rich foods can cause blood sugar levels to spike quickly, whereas protein and fiber-rich foods can help stabilize blood sugar levels.

2. Physical activity: Exercise can help the body use glucose more effectively, lowering blood sugar levels. Intense or prolonged exercise, on the other hand, can cause blood sugar levels to drop dangerously low.

3. Medications: Some medications, such as insulin and other diabetes medications, can have an immediate effect on blood sugar levels

.4. Illness or stress: Illness or stress can cause blood sugar levels to rise as stress hormones are released.

5. Sleep: Sleep deprivation or poor sleep quality can cause blood sugar levels to rise due to hormonal changes.

6. Hormones: Hormones such as insulin, glucagon, cortisol, and growth hormone play an important role in blood sugar regulation.

7. Age: As people get older, their bodies may become less sensitive to insulin, resulting in higher blood sugar levels.

8. Genetics: Some people may be genetically predisposed to developing diabetes or having difficulty regulating blood sugar levels.

Maintaining a healthy lifestyle, diet, regular exercise, and stress management are all important factors in controlling blood sugar levels. Individuals with diabetes or other conditions that affect blood sugar levels should also consult with a healthcare provider.

Glycemic Load and Glycemic Index

The glycemic index (GI) and glycemic load (GL) are two methods for determining how carbohydrate-containing foods affect blood sugar levels.

The glycemic index assigns a score of 0 to 100 to foods based on how quickly they raise blood sugar levels. Foods with a high GI (70 or higher) cause blood sugar levels to rise quickly, whereas foods with a low GI (55 or below) are digested more slowly and cause blood sugar levels to rise more slowly. Foods with a medium GI (56-69) are in the middle.

The glycemic load considers both the GI and the number of carbohydrates in food. It is calculated by multiplying the GI of a food by the carbohydrate content and then dividing by 100. Foods with a high GL (20 or higher) have a greater impact on blood sugar levels than foods with a low GL (10 or less).

High GI or GL foods can cause blood sugar levels to spike quickly, leading to a crash later on. This can be especially difficult for people who have diabetes or other conditions that affect blood sugar levels. Low GI or GL foods digest more slowly, resulting in a slower rise in blood sugar levels and more sustained energy levels.

It's important to remember that the GI and GL aren't the only things to think about when making food choices. Nutrient density, fiber content, and total calorie content are all important considerations. Understanding the glycemic index and glycemic load, on the other hand, can be a useful tool in making informed decisions about carbohydrate-containing foods.

The distinction between normal and high blood glucose levels

The amount of glucose in the blood is referred to as blood sugar levels, also known as blood glucose levels. Normal blood sugar levels fluctuate throughout the day depending on when and what you eat, but they generally fall within a certain range.

A normal blood sugar level for adults is typically between 70 and 100 mg/dL after an overnight fast of at least 8 hours (milligrams per deciliter). Blood sugar levels may temporarily rise after eating, but they should return to normal within a few hours.

High blood sugar levels, also known as hyperglycemia, occur when there is an excess of glucose in the blood. This can occur when Insulin resistance is a condition where the body produces insufficient insulin or when the body is resistant to insulin. Stress, illness, certain medications, and consuming too much food or liquid can all contribute to high blood sugar levels.

Increased thirst, frequent urination, blurred vision, fatigue, and headaches are all signs of high blood sugar. Long-term blood sugar levels that are too high can harm the blood vessels and nerves, which can result in complications like cardiovascular disease, kidney damage, and neuropathy.

To avoid the complications linked to high blood sugar levels, it's crucial to control blood sugar levels. This may entail making lifestyle adjustments like regular exercise, healthy eating, and weight management in addition to taking medication or receiving insulin therapy as directed by a doctor.

The dangers of having high blood sugar levels
Hyperglycemia, or high blood sugar levels, can lead to a variety of health issues. Here are some of the health risks associated with high blood sugar levels:

1. Diabetes: elevated levels of sugar in the blood are a defining feature of diabetes, a chronic disease that affects how the body processes sugar.

2. Cardiovascular disease: elevated levels of sugar in the blood can harm blood vessels, causing atherosclerosis, or plaque buildup in the arteries. This can increase the risk of developing heart disease, having a heart attack, or having a stroke.

3. Kidney damage: High blood sugar levels can harm the kidneys, causing diabetic nephropathy, which can eventually lead to kidney failure.

4. Vision loss: High blood sugar levels can damage the blood vessels in the eyes, resulting in diabetic retinopathy.

5. Neuropathy: High blood sugar levels can harm the body's nerves, causing a variety of symptoms such as pain, tingling, and numbness.

6. Foot issues: Diabetes can cause poor circulation and nerve damage in the feet, increasing the risk of foot ulcers and infections.

7. Slow wound healing: High blood sugar levels can stymie wound healing, increasing the risk of infection and complications.

To avoid these health issues, blood sugar levels must be controlled. This could include changes to one's lifestyle, such as regular exercise, healthy eating habits, and weight management. as well as any medication or insulin therapy prescribed by a physician.

Chapter 3

The Consequences of Poor Glucose Management,
Poor glucose management can have several short- and long-term consequences. The following are the immediate consequences:

1. Hypoglycemia:Low blood sugar levels can cause dizziness, confusion, weakness, and even unconsciousness.

2. Hyperglycemia:Excessive blood sugar levels can cause symptoms such as frequent urination, thirst, blurred vision, fatigue, and slow wound healing.

3. Diabetic ketoacidosis:This occurs when the body produces excessive amounts of ketones as a result of fat breakdown for energy when glucose is unavailable. It can cause nausea, vomiting, rapid breathing, and fruity-smelling breath.

Poor glucose management has the following long-term consequences:

1. Diabetes complications: Poor glucose management can lead to nerve damage, kidney disease, eye problems, cardiovascular disease, and poor circulation over time.

2. Infection risk: High blood sugar levels can weaken the immune system, increasing The danger of infections like urinary tract infections, pores and skin infections, and breathing infections.

3. Inadequate wound healing: High blood sugar levels can impair the body's ability to heal wounds, resulting in slower healing and an increased risk of infection.

4. Cognitive decline: High blood sugar levels can lead to cognitive decline and dementia over time. Overall, it is critical to maintain good glucose management to avoid both short-term and long-term consequences. This includes regularly monitoring blood sugar levels and taking medications as directed, eating a healthy diet and exercising regularly, and managing stress are all important.

Type 2 Diabetes and Insulin Resistance.

Insulin resistance is a circumstance wherein the cells of the frame come to be proof against the consequences of insulin, a hormone that aids in blood sugar regulation. As a result, to maintain normal blood sugar levels, the pancreas must produce more insulin, which can eventually lead to the development of type 2 diabetes. Type 2 diabetes is a chronic condition in which the body is unable to produce or use insulin effectively. High blood sugar levels can result, which can lead to a variety of health issues over time, including nerve damage, kidney damage, and cardiovascular disease.

Insulin resistance is a major risk factor for type 2 diabetes, and the two diseases are inextricably linked. Most people with type 2 diabetes have some level of insulin resistance. The body's ability to produce insulin can deteriorate over time, resulting in high blood sugar levels and the development of type 2 diabetes. Genetics, obesity, a lack of physical activity, and a poor diet are all factors that can contribute to the development of insulin resistance and type 2 diabetes. Both conditions are typically treated with lifestyle changes such as exercise, healthy eating, and weight management, as well as medications to help regulate blood sugar levels

Cardiovascular Illness.

A strong link exists between poor glucose management and cardiovascular disease (CVD). Diabetes, characterized by high blood sugar levels, is a significant risk factor for CVD. Diabetes patients are two to four times more likely than non-diabetics to develop CVD. Consistently high blood sugar levels can damage blood vessels, including the coronary arteries that supply blood to the heart. This increases the likelihood of plaque buildup, which can eventually lead to blockages and reduced blood flow to the heart, resulting in a heart attack. High blood sugar levels can also harm the nerves that control the heart, resulting in arrhythmias, or abnormal heart rhythms. Furthermore, high blood sugar levels can cause increased inflammation in the body, contributing to the development of CVD. As a result, maintaining healthy blood glucose levels is critical for the prevention and management of CVD, particularly in diabetics. This can be accomplished through lifestyle changes such as regular exercise, a healthy diet, blood sugar monitoring, and taking medications as prescribed by a healthcare provider. Syndrome Metabolique A metabolic syndrome is a group of conditions that occur in tandem and increase the likelihood of developing cardiovascular disease, stroke, and diabetes.

Metabolic syndrome

This is characterized by abdominal obesity, high blood pressure, elevated levels of blood sugar, high triglycerides, and low HDL cholesterol levels. A key feature of metabolic syndrome is poor glucose management. Individuals with metabolic syndrome, in particular, frequently have insulin resistance, which means their cells do not respond to insulin as well as they should. As a result, their pancreas must produce more insulin to help regulate blood sugar levels, which can eventually lead to elevated blood sugar levels. Hyperglycemia, or high blood sugar levels, can damage blood vessels and organs over time, resulting in complications such as nerve damage, kidney damage, and eye damage. Poor glucose management in people with metabolic syndrome is thus a serious health concern that should be managed and closely monitored through lifestyle changes and medical treatment.

Obesity and gaining weight

Obesity is a condition in which a person has too much body fat, which can be harmful to their health. Having a body mass index (BMI) of 30 or higher is considered obese. The BMI of a person is calculated by dividing their weight in kilograms by their height in meters squared. Weight gain can be caused by a variety of factors, including genetics, lifestyle, and environmental influences. When a person consumes more calories than they burn, the excess calories are stored as fat in the body, resulting in weight gain. Obesity can develop as a result of this over time.

Obesity and weight gain are linked to several health issues, including heart disease, type 2 diabetes, high blood pressure, sleep apnea, and certain cancers.

They are also linked to an increased risk of developing other conditions related to poor glucose management, such as metabolic syndrome, which is a collection of symptoms such as high blood pressure, high cholesterol, and high blood sugar levels. Metabolic syndrome can increase the risk of cardiovascular disease and stroke.

As a result, maintaining a healthy weight requires regular physical activity, healthy eating habits, and lifestyle changes.

If a person is struggling with obesity or weight gain, working with a healthcare professional or a registered dietitian to develop a personalized weight management plan may be beneficial. Setting realistic weight loss goals, increasing physical activity, and making dietary changes are all examples of this. Medication or surgery may be recommended as part of a comprehensive weight management plan in some cases.

Cognitive Impairment

Poor glucose management is linked to cognitive decline and an increased risk of developing conditions such as dementia and Alzheimer's disease, according to growing evidence.

High blood sugar levels can damage blood vessels and nerves in the brain, resulting in cognitive impairment. Furthermore, insulin resistance, which is common in people with poor glucose control, can impair the body's ability to break down and remove beta-amyloid protein, which is a key component of the plaques that form in the brains of people with Alzheimer's disease.

Studies have also shown that people with type 2 diabetes, which is frequently associated with poor glucose management, have a higher risk of developing dementia and Alzheimer's disease.

People with type 2 diabetes, which is often associated with poor glucose management, are also at a higher risk of developing dementia and Alzheimer's disease than those without diabetes, according to research. Furthermore, poor glucose management in middle age has been linked to a higher risk of diabetes/ higher risk of cognitive decline and dementia later in life.

Managing blood sugar levels through regular physical activity, healthy eating habits, and lifestyle changes may therefore help to reduce the risk of cognitive decline and related conditions. People with poor glucose management or diabetes may benefit from regular blood sugar monitoring and collaboration with healthcare professionals to effectively manage their condition.

Chapter 4

The Advantages of Intelligent Glucose Management

Smart glucose management can have a variety of health and well-being benefits, including:

Improved Athletic Performance

It can offer several advantages to athletes looking to improve their performance. Glucose management can help improve athletic performance in the following ways:

1. Increased Energy Levels: Proper glucose management can assist in maintaining consistent energy levels during workouts and competitions. Athletes can avoid energy crashes and maintain peak performance by maintaining stable blood glucose levels.

2. Improved Endurance: By ensuring that muscles have a steady supply of energy during exercise, glucose management can help improve endurance. This can help athletes perform at their peak for longer periods by delaying fatigue.

3. Faster Recovery: By replenishing glycogen stores in the muscles after exercise, glucose management can help improve recovery time. This can assist in reducing muscle soreness and allow athletes to bounce back faster after intense workouts or competitions.

4. Improved Cognitive Function: Because glucose is the brain's primary fuel source, maintaining stable glucose levels can help improve cognitive function, including focus and decision-making abilities. This is particularly important for athletes who must make split-second decisions during competitions.

5. Lowering the Risk of Injury: Smart glucose management can also help lower the risk of injury during exercise. Athletes can avoid energy crashes and dangerous drops in blood sugar levels by maintaining stable glucose levels, which can cause dizziness, confusion, and loss of coordination.

Improved Brain Function

Glucose is the brain's primary fuel source, and maintaining stable glucose levels can help improve cognitive function in a variety of ways:

1. Improved Focus and Attention: Glucose is necessary for brain function, and keeping glucose levels stable can help improve focus and attention. Low blood sugar levels have been linked to decreased cognitive function, including difficulty concentrating and poor memory, according to research.

2. Improved Decision-Making Ability: Diabetes management can also help improve decision-making abilities. The brain can function at its best when glucose levels are stable, allowing for better decision-making and problem-solving abilities.

3. Improved Mood: Smart glucose management may assist with mood improvement. Low blood sugar levels can trigger anxiety, mood swings, and exhaustion. People can experience greater energy and have a better overall sense of well-being by maintaining stable glucose levels.

4. Lower Risk of Cognitive Decline: Long-term glucose management has been shown in studies to help reduce the risk of cognitive decline and dementia. High blood sugar levels have been linked to an increased risk of Alzheimer's disease and other forms of dementia, making glucose management a critical component of brain health maintenance.

Increased Energy Levels

Glucose is the body's primary source of energy, and keeping glucose levels stable can help improve energy levels in a variety of ways:

1. Consistent Energy: By maintaining proper glucose levels, individuals can avoid energy crashes, which can cause fatigue and lethargy. Instead, they can maintain consistent energy levels throughout the day.

2. Increased Endurance: Smart glucose management can also aid in physical activity endurance. By making certain that muscles receive a constant supply of glucose. People can avoid fatigue and perform at their peak periods.

3. Quicker Recovery: Managing your glucose levels can also help you recover faster after physical activity. Individuals can reduce muscle soreness and recover faster after intense workouts by replenishing glycogen stores in the muscles.

4. Increased Mental Energy: Glucose is also necessary for brain function, and keeping glucose levels stable can help improve mental energy levels. This can result in improved focus, productivity, and mental clarity.

5. Lower Risk of Hypoglycemia: Hypoglycemia, or low blood sugar levels, can cause fatigue and lethargy.

Individuals can reduce their risk of hypoglycemia and enjoy consistent energy levels throughout the day by maintaining stable glucose levels.

In general, smart glucose management can be a useful tool for increasing energy levels. Individuals who maintain stable glucose levels can enjoy consistent energy levels throughout the day, improve endurance and recovery time during physical activity, and boost mental energy.

Anti-Aging and Longevity

Because high blood sugar levels are associated with an increased risk of chronic diseases and premature aging, glucose management is an important factor in maintaining overall health and well-being.

1. Lowering the Risk of Chronic Diseases: High blood sugar levels have been linked to an increased risk of chronic diseases like diabetes, heart disease, and certain types of cancer. Individuals can reduce their risk of these diseases and promote overall health and longevity by maintaining stable glucose levels.

2. Better Cellular Health: High blood sugar levels can cause cellular damage and inflammation, hastening the

aging process. Individuals can improve cellular health and slow the aging process by maintaining stable glucose levels.

3. Improved Skin Health: High blood sugar levels can damage collagen and elastin, causing wrinkles and other aging signs. Individuals can promote better skin health and reduce the signs of aging by maintaining stable glucose levels.

4. Improved Cognitive Function: Diabetes has been linked to cognitive decline and dementia. People can enhance cognitive function and reduce the risk of age-related cognitive impairment by maintaining stable glucose levels.

5. Increased Longevity: Studies have shown that people who keep their glucose levels stable throughout their lives live longer and have better overall health and well-being.

Chapter 5

Glucose Management Strategies

Managing glucose levels is critical for overall health, especially for people with diabetes or pre-diabetes. Here are some glucose management strategies:

Dietary Methods

A dietary approach is a specific way of eating that is designed to achieve specific health objectives. There are various dietary approaches, each with its own philosophy and food recommendations.

Among the most common dietary approaches are:

1. The Mediterranean diet This diet emphasizes fruits and vegetables, whole grains, legumes, nuts and seeds, and healthy fats such as olive oil while limiting red meat, sugar, and processed foods.

2. Low-carbohydrate diet: This method restricts carbohydrates such as grains, sugars, and starchy vegetables while emphasizing protein and healthy fats such as nuts, seeds, avocados, and olive oil.

3. Plant-based diet: This diet emphasizes plant foods such as fruits and vegetables, whole grains, legumes, nuts, and seeds while limiting or eliminating animal products.

4. Dash diet: This diet emphasizes whole foods such as fruits and vegetables, whole grains, low-fat dairy, lean proteins, and healthy fats while limiting sodium and processed foods.

5. Paleo diet: This way of eating emphasizes whole, unprocessed foods such as meat, fish, eggs, fruits, vegetables, nuts, and seeds while avoiding grains, legumes, and dairy.

It's important to remember that there is no one-size-fits-all diet, and the best diet for an individual is determined by a variety of factors such as health status, age, activity level, and personal preferences. A healthcare professional or a registered dietitian can assist an individual in determining the best dietary approach.

Physical Activity and Exercising

Physical activity and exercise are essential for maintaining a healthy body and mind. Exercise is any planned, structured, and repetitive physical activity, whereas physical activity is any movement that requires energy expenditure. Physical activity and exercise can both improve overall health and lower the risk of chronic diseases.

• Increases muscle strength and endurance

- Improves cardiovascular health
- Aids in weight management
- Improves flexibility and balance
- Reduces stress and anxiety
- Promotes better sleep
- Improves cognitive function
- Boosts mood and self-esteem
- Aerobic exercises, such as running, cycling, or swimming, involves the continuous movement of large muscle groups.
- Strength training, such as weightlifting, involves using resistance to build muscle mass and increase strength.
- Flexibility training consists of stretching exercises designed to increase the range of motion and prevent injury.
- Balance training consists of exercises designed to improve stability and prevent falls.

Walking, gardening, and doing household chores are all examples of physical activity. It is recommended that you engage in at least 150 minutes of moderate-intensity physical activity per week or 75 minutes of vigorous-intensity physical activity per week, as well as muscle-strengthening activities at least twice a week.

Before beginning any exercise program, it is critical to consult with a healthcare provider, especially if you have any health conditions or injuries.

Changes in Lifestyle

Managing glucose levels is critical for diabetics, and making lifestyle changes can be an effective strategy for accomplishing this goal. Here are some lifestyle changes that can aid in glucose management:

1. Consuming a well-balanced diet: Consuming a well-balanced diet rich in complex carbohydrates, protein, healthy fats, and fiber can help regulate glucose levels. It's also important to avoid simple carbohydrates like sugary drinks and processed foods.

2. Regular physical activity: By improving insulin sensitivity and promoting weight loss, regular physical activity can help lower glucose levels. On most days of the week, aim for at least 30 minutes of moderate-intensity exercise.

3. Maintaining a healthy weight: Excess weight can impair the body's ability to use insulin properly, resulting in high glucose levels. Weight loss through a combination of diet and exercise can aid in glucose control.

4. Regular glucose monitoring: Regular glucose monitoring can help people with diabetes identify patterns and make necessary changes to their diet and medication.

5. Stress management: Stress causes the body to release hormones that raise glucose levels. Finding healthy ways to manage stress, such as meditation or exercise, can aid in glucose control.

6. Get enough sleep: Sleep deprivation can increase insulin resistance, leading to high glucose levels. Each night, aim for seven to eight hours of sleep.

7. Quitting smoking: Smoking can make it difficult to control glucose levels and increase the risk of diabetes complications. Smoking cessation can improve overall health and lower the risk of complications.

These lifestyle changes can be difficult to implement, but working with a healthcare provider or a registered dietitian can assist people with diabetes in developing a plan that works for them.

Supplements for Nutrition

To manage glucose levels in diabetics, nutritional supplements may be used in addition to lifestyle changes and medication. However, before taking any nutritional supplements, consult with a healthcare provider because some supplements may interact with medications or have negative effects on health. Here are some nutritional supplements that may help with glucose management:

1. Chromium: Chromium is a mineral that aids the body's use of insulin. Some research suggests that chromium supplementation may improve glucose control in diabetics. However, the evidence is conflicting, and more research is required.

2. Magnesium: Magnesium is a mineral that aids in the metabolism of glucose. According to research, magnesium supplementation may improve glucose control in diabetics, particularly those who are magnesium deficient.

3. Alpha-lipoic acid: Alpha-lipoic acid is an antioxidant that may aid in glucose control and the reduction of diabetic neuropathy symptoms. More research, however, is required to determine its effectiveness.

4. Vitamin D: Vitamin D is important for insulin sensitivity, and low vitamin D levels have been linked to an increased risk of diabetes. Some research suggests that vitamin D supplementation may improve glucose control in diabetics.

5. Probiotics: Probiotics are beneficial bacteria that live in the gastrointestinal tract. According to some studies, probiotic supplementation may improve glucose control in individuals with diabetes, although the evidence is mixed.

It's important to remember that nutritional supplements aren't a replacement for a healthy diet and lifestyle changes, and they should be used in conjunction with them. Furthermore, not all supplements are safe or effective, and some may cause adverse effects. Before taking any nutritional supplements, always consult with your doctor.

Chapter 6

Putting Your Glucose Management Plan into Action

Implementing a glucose management plan can be difficult, but diabetics must maintain healthy glucose levels and avoid complications.

Here are some steps to help you put your glucose management plan into action:

-Develop specific objectives: Set realistic goals for your glucose management plan with your healthcare provider. Your objectives should be specific, measurable, attainable, timely, and relevant (SMART). SMART goals for glucose management could include lowering your HbA1c levels by a certain percentage or reaching a certain fasting blood glucose level.

-

Create an action plan: Once you've determined your objectives, create a detailed action plan outlining the steps you'll take to achieve them. Dietary changes, increased physical activity, medication adjustments, or a combination of these strategies may be included in this plan. Work with your healthcare provider to ensure that your plan is both safe and effective.

-Track your progress: It is critical to regularly monitor your blood glucose levels and track your progress toward your goals to stay on track. To track your glucose levels throughout the day, consider using a blood glucose monitor or a continuous glucose monitoring (CGM) device. You should also keep a log of your food intake, physical activity, and medication use to help identify patterns and make necessary adjustments.

Adjust your plan as needed: As you track your progress, be ready to make changes to your plan as necessary. If you are not making progress towards your goals, discuss potential adjustments with your healthcare provider. Changes to your medication regimen, diet, or exercise routine may be included.

-Celebrate your accomplishments: Finally, remember to celebrate your accomplishments along the way. Even small victories can add up, and acknowledging your progress can keep you motivated to continue making positive changes in your glucose management plan.

Chapter 7

Conclusion

The Future of Glucose Control

Technological and research advances are likely to shape the future of glucose management. Here are some potential developments that could impact glucose management in the future.

1. Continuous glucose monitoring (CGM): CGM devices are already available, but they are likely to become more widespread and accurate in the future. People with diabetes can use this technology to monitor their glucose levels in real-time and make informed decisions about diet, exercise, and medication.

2. Artificial pancreas: An artificial pancreas is a closed-loop system that uses a CGM device and insulin pump to automatically adjust insulin dosing based on glucose levels. This technology is still in development, but it has the potential to revolutionize glucose management for diabetics.

3. Gene editing: Scientists are investigating the possibility of using gene editing to treat diabetes by modifying genes

involved in glucose metabolism. While this technology is still in its infancy, it has the potential to provide a long-term cure for diabetes.

4. Personalized medicine: Advances in genetics and personalized medicine may result in diabetes treatments that are tailored to an individual's genetic makeup and other factors.

5. Lifestyle interventions: Lifestyle interventions, such as dietary changes and exercise, can help manage glucose levels significantly. The technology could be used in the future to create personalized lifestyle interventions based on an individual's needs and preferences.
Overall, the future of glucose management will most likely involve a combination of technology and personalized medicine, with a focus on preventing complications and improving people with diabetes quality of life.

The potential impact of these innovations on diabetes and other glucose disorders treatment

The innovations mentioned earlier have the potential to revolutionize the treatment of diabetes and other glucose disorders in several ways:

1. Improved glucose control: Continuous glucose monitoring and the artificial pancreas could help people with diabetes achieve better glucose control, reducing the risk of complications such as neuropathy, retinopathy, and kidney disease.

2. Increased convenience: The use of technology such as CGM devices and insulin pumps can provide increased convenience for people with diabetes, allowing them to manage their condition more easily while going about their daily lives.

3. More personalized treatment: Advances in genetics and personalized medicine may lead to tailored diabetes treatments based on an individual's genetic makeup and other factors, potentially improving outcomes and reducing the need for trial and error in determining the most effective treatment.

4. Prevention of complications: The earlier detection and management of glucose disorders made possible by these innovations could prevent or delay the onset of

complications associated with diabetes, improving quality of life and reducing healthcare costs.

5. A potential cure: Gene editing could eventually provide a long-term cure for diabetes, eliminating the need for ongoing management of the condition.

Overall, these innovations have the potential to significantly improve the treatment and management of diabetes and other glucose disorders, providing greater convenience, better outcomes, and potentially even a cure for this chronic condition.

Appendix

Recipes and Meal Plans for Managing Blood Sugar

Here are some suggestions and ideas to keep in mind if you're looking for recipes and meal plans to help manage glucose levels:

1. Emphasize whole, nutritious foods: Prioritize whole, nutrient-dense foods like vegetables, fruits, lean proteins, healthy fats, and whole grains instead of relying on processed foods or meals high in refined carbohydrates.

2. Aim for balanced meals: A balanced diet that includes a variety of protein, healthy fats, and fiber-rich carbohydrates can help to stabilize blood sugar levels by reducing the rate at which glucose is absorbed into the body.

3. Take into account portion sizes: Even though whole foods are typically a good choice, eating too much can still result in high glucose levels. Pay close attention to portion sizes and make an effort to balance the intake of various food groups.

4. Space out meals throughout the day: Eating smaller, more frequent meals can assist in maintaining stable

blood sugar levels all day long. Aim for three meals and two snacks per day, or however often you feel most satiated by eating.

5. Stay hydrated: Dehydration can result in higher glucose levels, so drinking plenty of water can help maintain stable blood sugar levels.

Here are some menu plans and recipe suggestions:

BREAKFAST:

• Eggs scrambled with avocado and spinach
• Greek yogurt topped with a variety of berries and a dash of nuts or seeds
• Overnight oats with chia seeds, berries, and almond milk

Lunch:

consists of a grilled chicken salad with mixed greens, tomatoes, cucumbers, and vinaigrette dressing.
• Quinoa bowl with roasted vegetables and tahini dressing
• Tuna salad with sliced vegetables and whole grain crackers

Dinner:

 baked chicken thighs with roasted Brussels sprouts and brown rice, grilled salmon with sweet potatoes and broccoli, lentil soup with mixed vegetables, and a side salad.

SNACKS include cheese and whole grain crackers, carrots, hummus, and sliced apples with almond butter.

Keep in mind that each person has unique requirements for managing their blood sugar, so it's crucial to collaborate with a healthcare professional to create a tailored strategy.

www.ingramcontent.com/pod-product-compliance
Lightning Source LLC
Chambersburg PA
CBHW061606250726

48657CB00017B/2200